Becoming Bulle

An Uncommon Approach to Building a Resilient Body

by
Tim Anderson and
Mike McNiff

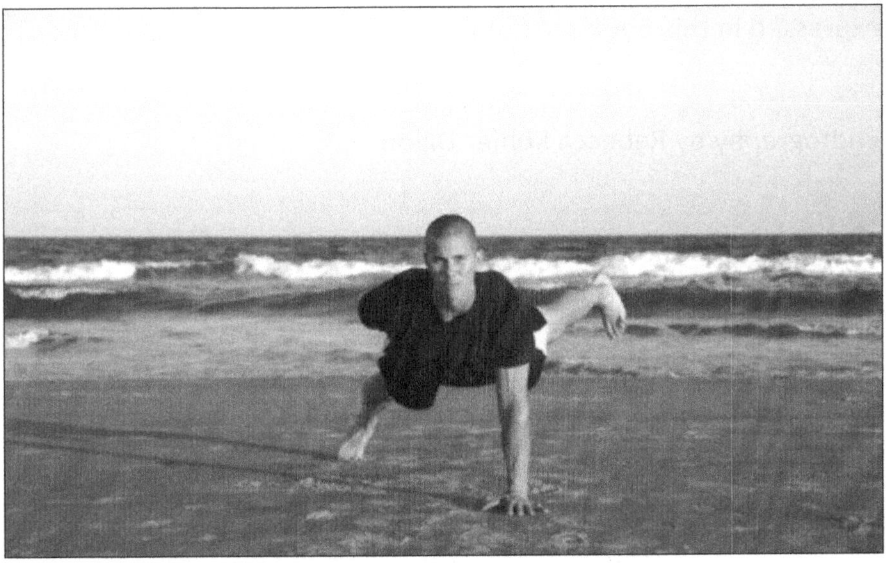

xulon PRESS

Becoming Bulletproof
An Uncommon Approach to Building a Resilient Body
by Tim Anderson and Mike McNiff

Printed in the United States of America

ISBN 9781619961968

Photography by Rebecca Kohler Dillon

www.xulonpress.com

Special Thanks

We would like to thank God first. The journey that led to the writing of this book was nothing short of divine. God has had his hand in this every step of the way. For that, we are grateful and humbled. Thank you, Lord.

Thank you Geoff and Courtney Neupert for listening to us and supporting us with our ideas. We appreciate your friendship and your help.

From Mike:

I would like to thank my best friend Tim for believing in me when I had given up hope and my two daughters, Britney and Cameron, for giving me a reason to be strong.

From Tim:

Thanks to my wife, Addie, for putting up with me and listening to me for 18 wonderful years even though I drive you completely crazy. I love you.

Thanks to Mike, my new brother from another mother. It has been a great journey and it is only just beginning.

Thanks to my mentor, John Brookfield. You have been a fountain of wisdom and guidance for me, and I can never thank you enough.

Table of Contents

Becoming Bulletproof

This book is about becoming bulletproof. We guess this is a good time to explain what we mean when we say *bulletproof*. The body should be capable of doing anything without limitations. We should be able to run, jump and play without sustaining nagging injuries or acquiring other "movement issues." The body is made to be powerful, durable and resilient. When we are 70 years old, our bodies should still have all of these qualities. Simply put, being bulletproof means having a healthy body that allows us to enjoy life well into our golden years. It means having a body free from pain, restrictions and limitations.

This book is a collaborative effort that started from conversations Mike and I had about training. We were both searching for ways to unlock our bodies' potential and overcome our own movement issues and limitations. What we found, through our conversations, research and application has further cemented the idea that we were made to be bulletproof. After all, we are fearfully and wonderfully made.

Life should be about being happy. If you really want to be happy, you need a healthy body. Being in pain and always being injured should not be the norm or the status quo. We should be able to go for a run without getting knee pain. We should be able to pick up a suitcase without hurting our backs. We should be able to grab something out of the back seat of our car without tearing a rotator cuff. We should be resilient! We were not meant to be fragile.

We believe the information in this book will truly help you press the "reset button" on your body and help you rebuild the body you were meant to have: a strong, flexible, powerful body capable of climbing any mountain or swimming any sea. We invite you to engage in your own journey and learn how to become resilient and unlock your full potential. Regain the body you were meant to have.

You were meant to be bulletproof.

Life is Movement

The writing has been on the wall all along. Movement is the key to becoming bulletproof. Even before we are born we start developing our brains and bodies through movement.[1] Once we are born, we build a huge movement foundation and movement vocabulary through movement patterns like lifting our heads, rolling, creeping and crawling. At the same time these movements are developing our bodies, they are also developing our brains. In *The Well Balanced Child,* Ewout Van-Manen points out that "... physical movement is the basis for cognitive, social and emotional development."[2]

What does all of this have to do with becoming bulletproof? Everything! Becoming bulletproof is not just physical. Brain development is not mutually exclusive from body development. The better you move, the better your brain functions and vice-versa.

Our bodies were meant to move in all possible combinations of movements and in all planes of motion. We are designed to be physically capable of anything. From the moment we are born, we begin learning and earning our movement abilities. We develop our movement foundation by exploring the world through our senses and learning how to move our bodies. Through movement, we develop our "body map", our sense of self in space. This is called proprioception.[3] Our body is filled with sensors, and proprioceptors, that feed our brain with a sense of self every time we move and experience our environment. The more we move, the more clear our body map becomes. The clearer our body map is, the better we move.

Dr. Eric Cobb, creator of the Z-health Performance System, uses a good analogy to illustrate this. He says to imagine your brain holds a 3D map of your body. In order to have a good map, you have to have good information. If the 3D map is fuzzy, you may not have good information from your nerves, i.e., you may not move so well. If you are getting good information from all the proprioceptors in your skin, joints, tendons and muscles, your movement map will be quite clear. If you are not getting good information from your proprioceptors, your movement map may be fuzzy.

Not only does movement improve your proprioception, it actually physically changes and improves your brain! Physical activity develops brain tissue![4] Inside your brain, there are millions of nerve connections, or nerve networks. Movement improves the communication between these connections and cements new connections.[5] The better you move, the more efficient your brain becomes. The more efficient your brain becomes, the better you move. It's a two-way street.

Movement truly is life. It shapes everything about us: our brains, our bodies, who we are as people, our emotions, our hormones, even our mental health.[6] Movement is the key to health; every facet of health. BUT, by the age of five, we do something very unnatural; we learn to sit six to eight hours a day while we begin "learning" in school. Movement, the very thing that shapes our brains and our life, is halted so we can begin to shape our brains through our wonderful education process. The movements and patterns we developed as a child are suddenly put aside and we learn a new pattern: sitting. We spend years sitting: over a computer, in a car, in a chair, on the couch. We have become very, very good at sitting. We get so good at sitting we become stuck in the seated position, or the "adult fetal position," because all of our flexor muscles become so tight. We are not designed to sit still for six to eight hours everyday, or any day. It is not natural.

The ironic thing is we all know we should stay fit and healthy so we go to the local fitness center that allows us to "train" and workout while we are sitting down! Do you want to know how to make a movement pattern stick, good or bad? Load it with weight. Yes, we go to the health club, sit down on a machine and lift a weight or ride a bike. We cement our ability to sit by exercising in the seated position, and we further lose our ability to be bulletproof!

We are made to move. Yet, most of us don't move. We sit instead. So, we lose our movement patterns, or we replace them with sitting. We slow our brain development. In some ways, our brain development regresses. This process is called neuronal fitness or neuronal pruning.[7] Just as movement can shape and develop our brains, not moving can also shape our brains. Simply put, our brains prune out the nerve connections we don't need or the ones we don't use often. The neural connections in the brain are much like the movement patterns in the body: **use it or lose it.**

We live in a world filled with technological innovations and conveniences. We have computers, we have cars, we have the internet. There is no need for us to get up and move. If we want to go shopping, we only have to jump online. We don't even have to get out and go to the mall anymore! Every year we grow further and further away from physical bodies capable of anything to bodies capable of being paper weights. We are wonderfully made, yet we don't allow ourselves to participate in the wonder for which we were created. We were made to move, anywhere and everywhere. Yet most of us spend our time going nowhere. That is to say, we occupy the same square footage of a chair for hours and hours every day. Many kids are not even learning how to run, how to skip, or how to climb. We are moving further and further away from what we were made for: movement. Remember, movement is life, *and* life is movement!

There are some things we cannot change. Kids have to go to school, adults have to go to work. In today's world we are going to spend a lot of time sitting. However, that doesn't mean we can't learn to minimize the time we spend sitting, and it doesn't mean we can't keep our bodies fit and capable of doing anything. We can learn to move deliberately. We can regain our movement patterns and get rid of our movement limitations. We can become healthy and resilient.

Most of the information in this book has been well researched and applied in the areas of learning disabilities, brain development and brain rehabilitation. We are extrapolating from these ideas used for building a healthy brain and applying this information, along with our own ideas, towards building a healthy body. After all, it takes a healthy body to build a healthy brain, and it takes a healthy brain to build a healthy body. The two are not mutually exclusive!

The 3D X

It is all about the center. One of the keys to becoming bulletproof is to have a fully functioning, reflexively stable, solid center. Yes, a strong core like you've heard for years! BUT a strong core is not something you get from doing abdominal exercises. A strong core is something that you earn when you are a developing child. It is comprised of not only muscles but reflexes, proprioceptive information from nerve signals, and movement patterns. A solid core is built by moving the way we were designed to move in all planes of motion. A child develops a fully functioning center by exploring movement and fully integrating movement with his or her senses. We are fully integrated. Our palms, our feet, our necks, our vestibular system (our balance system), our movement patterns - they all work together to develop our center. Take away one facet of our body (like wearing thick shoes all your life), or try to isolate one system from another, and we will weaken our core. Everything together makes the whole!

To understand the importance of a fully functioning center, it may help to think of our bodies as being an X (because our body is an X!). Not only are we shaped like one big X, but our entire body is made up of a series of Xs. Just look at an anatomy chart of muscles and notice how the muscles and tendons lie in relation to one another. Even our DNA is in the shape of a double helix, a spiraling X. We are literally a series of connected Xs from head to toe. The center of our X, our core, is where the forces we generate from movement cross over from one side of our body to the other. These forces cross through our center from left to right, right to left, bottom to top, and top to bottom. The more "connected" our X is, the more efficient the forces can cross over. We are made to be efficient and powerful.

Our center is not a two dimensional X. It is three dimensional, more like a tightly woven Chinese finger trap, or an hour glass that runs from the knees to the arm pits. Yes, the core is not just the midsection, but rather the mid torso. Paul Check, renowned expert in the field of high performance exercise kinesiology and founder of the CHEK Institute, uses a good description of our core as having an inner unit and an outer unit. However you view the core, it is the crossroads of force production. When everything is working as it should, the core is the crossroads of efficient and powerful forces; the key to a strong and resilient body.[8] When things in the core are not functioning properly, the core can be the crossroads of energy chaos; forces end up going in areas they shouldn't, creating stresses and energy leakages. In other words, if your center, or your core, is not functioning properly, you will not be as powerful as you were meant to be, and you may be at a higher risk of injury.

The vestibular system, or the balance system, is tied to the core. [9] Your grip is tied to your core. Your feet are tied to your core. Your skin is tied to your core. Your emotions are even tied to your core. Your core is tied to **EVERYTHING**. It all works together. Nothing is isolated. Everything is integrated.

Unfortunately, we are really good at isolating things that should not be isolated. We create conveniences in life that allow us to be comfortable so we don't have to move. Things like chairs, rear view mirrors, computers, remote controls, etc. We have gotten really good at not moving our heads or our bodies. We have become masters of disintegration. In return, we lose some of our movement patterns, we stagnate our vestibular system, we lose our reflexively stable core, and we become broken. We lose these things not simply because we do not use them but because we do not need them with our current lifestyles. As Mike likes to say, "We have tried to outsmart what we were designed to do."

So how do you go about fixing the imbalances and developing a strong "core" as an adult? By following the same developmental strategies that were in place for you as a child. We truly believe if we want to become physically resilient, we need to do what babies do; earn our strength and mobility through movement (some very *particular* movements that we will examine later).

But, before we examine those particular movements, lets take a closer look at the vestibular system, and see how it may be the key to building that reflexively strong core, the 3D X.

The Vestibular System

The vestibular system, which provides your sense of balance, directly affects your movement patterns and your ability to develop a strong core. It may be the most important sensory system you have, shaping everything about you: your sense of self, your reality, your balance, your posture, your ability to learn, your experiences, everything.[10] You can function without other sensory systems and lead a somewhat "normal" life. For instance, a blind man can learn to be independent and get around almost as well as people who have sight. But a person who's vestibular system is out of whack may not be able to have a "normal" life. Just ask anyone who has ever had vertigo and they will tell you just how important a healthy vestibular system is for feeling "normal" and healthy.

The vestibular system lives in your head, or your inner ears. It is composed of highly sensitive organs called the utricle, saccule, and semicircular canals.[11] Without getting too scientific, they are like having your own internal gyroscopes inside your head. The organs are filled with tiny hairs and a gel-like substance. When your head moves, the liquid substance moves the tiny hairs and sends information to your brain. Basically, they work to give you equilibrium and balance.[12]

The vestibular system is the first system to begin developing in the womb. It begins developing about 21 days after conception,[13] and it is fully developed about 5 months after conception.[14] Even in the womb, the mother's movements provide stimulation to the developing vestibular system. This stimulation helps develop the child's nervous system. Once a child is born, the new world of gravity and all the challenges it brings begin to further stimulate the vestibular system and shape the nervous system with the new movements the child begins to make.

The vestibular system may be the "King of the Senses" because everything is tied to it. Your proprioceptive system, or your inner sense of self and all your senses, is intimately tied to your vestibular system.[15] Together, they form your body map, or your movement map. The vestibular system is also connected to every muscle in your body, especially the core and neck muscles![16] Even your emotions can be affected by your vestibular system.[17] The vestibular system seems to be the foundational system that the rest of "you" is built upon.

A healthy vestibular system is crucial to having a healthy body. The more we move, the more we stimulate our vestibular system. The more we stimulate our vestibular system, the more nerve connections we make in our brain and our body. It has even been shown that children who receive regular vestibular stimulation show advanced development in motor skills.[18] Remember, all your muscles are tied to your vestibular system. If we continually stimulate our vestibular system, we continually stimulate all of our muscles in some way, especially our core and neck muscles.

When we don't move, we are not stimulating the vestibular system. In other words, we are not stimulating the brain, the nervous system, or the muscular system. Think of it this way, everything about the body follows the rule, "use it or lose it." The vestibular system is no different. If we do not train one of our most important senses or systems, perhaps the most important system we have, it will begin to deteriorate much like our calculus skills slip away after we get out of college. Sally Goddard Blythe points out that one of the first signs of brain deterioration is when balance starts to deteriorate.[19] If your vestibular system is indeed connected to every muscle in your body, your ability to move well will also deteriorate when your vestibular system deteriorates.

This is important: The vestibular system is tied to the core musculature of the abdominals and back, and it is these muscles that first work together to move the head.[20] The vestibular system is stimulated by neck movement, among other things. Moving the neck and head is tied to your core musculature. When a child picks up his head while lying on the floor, he is developing his core and training his vestibular system. They are not mutually exclusive.

It is **our belief** that when we sit all day and keep our heads still without moving our necks, we are detraining and weakening our core. Again, this is our hypothesis, but it makes a ton of sense. The human body is designed to move. Every system, every facet of the body is fully integrated. There is nothing about the body that is mutually exclusive from another part of itself. So, **EVERYTHING** about you is tied together in some way. You want to get a strong core? Start moving. Start moving your neck, start stimulating your vestibular system.

To recap, we believe the secret to a strong body is a strong center. If your core muscles are tied to your vestibular system, it only makes sense that a healthy vestibular system is crucial to having a strong center (3D X). The healthier our vestibular system is, the healthier and more resilient our bodies will become.

So, how do we train our vestibular system and develop a strong core? We move! We run, we jump, we spin, we roll, we flip, we rock. We do anything but sit in a chair for most of the day while we try to keep our heads still.

In fact, we believe there are certain moves that can "reset" the body and stimulate the vestibular system with a proprioceptive flood of information. In other words, we believe we can press "reset" with certain movements to regain, and re-earn, the body we were meant to have.

In the next four chapters, we will explore these movements, along with some other reflexes, that we believe will help you press “reset” and become bulletproof.

Pressing "Reset"

Two halves make a whole. Your brain has two hemispheres, the right hemisphere, or the gestalt side, and the left hemisphere, or the logic side. For your body to be efficient at anything, both hemispheres need to work together.[21] Performing midline crossing movements, also known as cross-lateral movements, seems to increase the communication between the two hemispheres.[22] Midline crossing movements can actually cause the brain to make new neural connections between the two hemispheres. This is what makes midline crossing movements crucial for learning and brain development. We believe it is also what makes them crucial for physical development. The more neural connections between the two hemispheres, the better the hemispheres work together and communicate with the body (i.e. the better you move).

Midline crossing movements are movements like crawling, running, skipping, and walking. In these movements, the opposite arm moves with the opposite leg in a coordinated motion, *usually* to get you from one point to another point. The first midline crossing movement we would like to introduce to you is known as the cross-crawl. It is a phenomenal tool for making the brain and body more efficient.

Cross-crawls are a midline crossing movement where you take the opposite hand, or elbow, and touch it to the opposite knee.[23] They can be done sitting, standing, or lying down. The magic behind cross crawls is that they activate large areas of both hemispheres of the brain simultaneously.[24] And, when done on a regular, consistent basis, they actually improve the neural connections between the hemispheres, allowing for faster communication between the hemispheres and better communication between the brain and the body.[25] Cross crawls have even been instrumental in successfully helping patients recover from strokes and helping children overcome ADD and ADHD.[26]

Cross-crawling encourages better neural connections and even new nerve cell growth in the brain! And, you don't have to have a learning disability or a stroke to perform them. Anyone can improve their brain function and their body with cross-crawls because the healthier the brain becomes, the healthier the body becomes. This simple movement highlights the statement that movement is life.

Crawling is another midline crossing movement that **most** of us should have done as a child. Research has shown that those who skip crawling are more likely to have learning disorders.[27] They are more likely to have movement and coordination issues as well because crawling sets the foundation for gait. The beautiful thing about crawling is that you don't have to be a baby to do it. Anyone can learn how to crawl.

Though similar to cross-crawls, crawling offers other benefits as well. Through mechanoreceptors, nerve endings, in the hands and feet, crawling stimulates reflexive core musculature activation, which gets the shoulders and pelvis working together.[28]

Crawling can also improve your binocular vision, your hand-eye coordination, and even your binaural hearing (your perception of sound from two ears).[29] In *The Well Balanced*

Child, Sally Goddard Blythe points out that "Movement on all fours also helps to align the spine at the back of the neck with the sacral region in preparation for proper alignment in the upright posture."[30] Crawling helps lay the foundation, on multiple levels, of who we become. In our discussions about becoming bulletproof, Mike said that "We are simply trying to outsmart what we were designed to do." Mike is a genius! How many parents like to brag about how fast their kids learn to walk? How many parents try to hasten the process by putting their kids in walkers or other contraptions to encourage walking? We were meant to crawl, and with good reason. In today's world, crawling should probably be done by everyone, everyday, young and old alike. It can be a great tool for building a resilient, capable body.

I know what you're thinking: *But babies learn to crawl so they can walk. We were made and designed to walk on two feet. Babies progress to walking! We are not supposed to keep crawling around as adults!*

You're absolutely right! **But**, we're not supposed to sit around all day either. And yet, that is what most of us do. Yes, walking and running are both a mid-line crossing movement that require coordination and they should incorporate both hemispheres of our brains. But, you know what? **You can fake walking and running.** You can walk and run without using your shoulders and arms properly. You can even do it without using them at all. **You cannot fake crawling.** It is deliberate. Your shoulders and hips have to work together. With crawling, they are both working together under load. Crawling sets things right, the way they were meant to be. It is the foundation, the template, for our gait pattern. Crawling is the ultimate "reset" pattern. It helps keep our 3D X, our center, functioning properly.

As great as crawling is, we have found that some clients just cannot crawl well; they have zero coordination. We have also had other clients that just didn't seem to get as big of a bang for their buck from crawling. Turns out, crawling is not the first thing we start doing when we start learning how to move. We rock before we crawl. We roll before we rock. And, we raise our heads before we roll. Some people, maybe all people, should spend some time rocking and rolling! Others should spend some time learning how to move their necks and stimulating their vestibular system.

Gray Cook has a DVD called *Secrets of the Primitive Patterns.* In discussing movement issues, he states that you can fix a lot of issues by correcting primitive patterns.[31]

Rolling is a primitive pattern. It is how most of us first learn to traverse the floor as babies. Rolling stimulates the vestibular system in a big way. (Remember, the vestibular system is tied to the core muscles.) Rolling also helps us develop rotary trunk stability. It prepares us for gait; crawling, walking, and running. We have witnessed rolling address several movement issues in clients. (These movement issues were revealed by using Gray Cook's Functional Movement Screen - The FMS). We have also witnessed dramatic improvements in strength, movement efficiency, stability, endurance and resiliency thanks to teaching clients how to roll.

Rocking is another primitive pattern. Rocking, or Quadruped Rocking, prepares the body for crawling. Not only that, it seems to really help with pelvic and scapular stabilization, and it may help align the spine.[32] Basically, rocking is a great way to start tying the core / body together. Rocking is done by getting on your hands and knees, keeping a long spine (chest up!) and rocking your butt back towards your calves. This drill can unlock a world of movement function for people. Rocking is also good for opening up the hips and it seems to help develop good posture.

Rolling, rocking, crawling, and cross crawling are all great tools for pressing the "reset button" for the body. Using the Functional Movement Screen (FMS)[33] as an assessment tool for our clients, we have found that these midline crossing movements have been great for restoring movement patterns, addressing asymmetries and correcting other movement issues. They have even helped some of our clients with some instances of pain. If you want to get your body functioning like it was meant to and you want to become fully connected and integrated, in every sense, these movements work wonders.

Dan John, a famous strength coach and author, taught me (Tim) a very valuable lesson:

If something is important, you should do it everyday.[34]

These four movements are important. **Do** them everyday. It all adds up, they can truly help unlock your potential and put you on your way to becoming bulletproof.

How To Press "Reset"

Before we get too deep in our progressions for becoming bulletproof, it may be a good idea to learn how to press the reset button. After all, we have to crawl before we walk!

How to Cross-Crawl

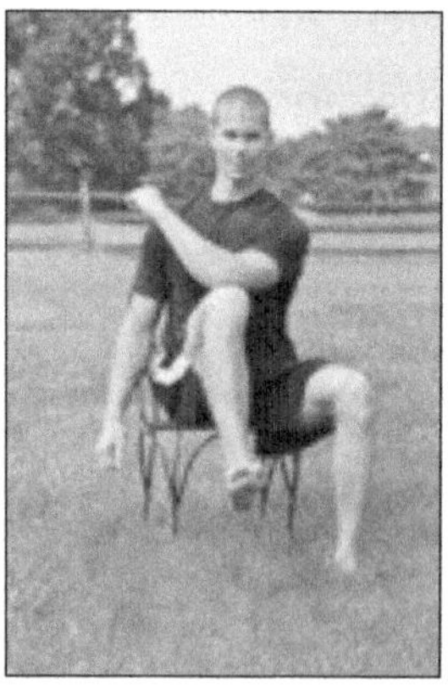

Seated Cross-Crawl

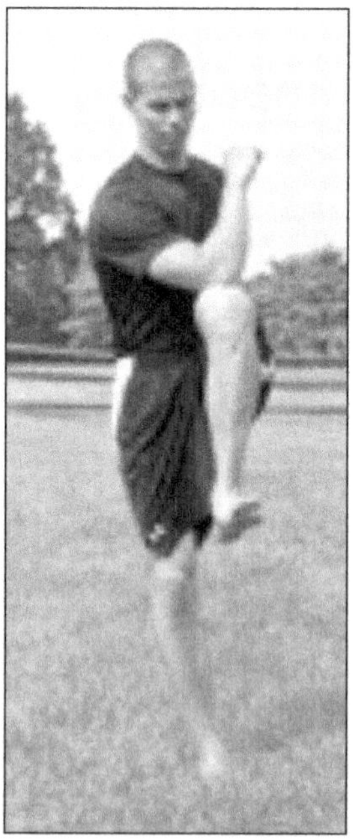

Standing Cross-Crawl

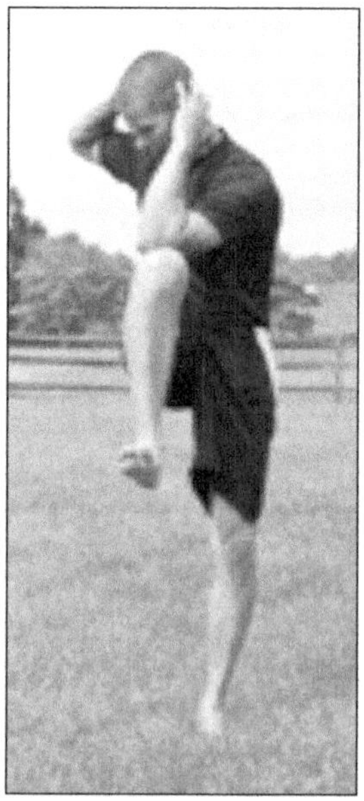

Fingers Behind Ears

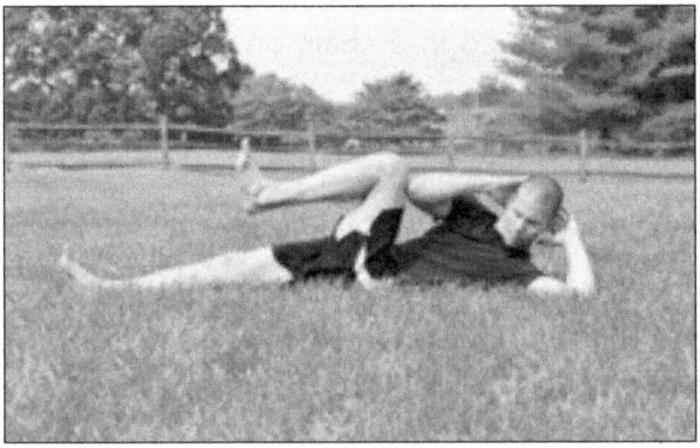

Lying Cross-Crawl

Cross-crawls are nothing new. You've probably even done them before in gym class. Athletes have been using them off and on for years as part of a warm-up routine. Chiropractors like Dr. Leroy Perry, the first chiropractor ever to serve as an Olympic Team Doctor, have always known that they benefit the body. But for some reason, cross-crawls have really only been recognized for how they benefit the brain, not so much for how they benefit the body physically. Remember, if you benefit one, you benefit the other!

A cross-crawl is done by walking in place while touching your opposite elbow to your opposite knee. In doing so, you are crossing mid-line of the body and activating both hemispheres of your brain with the coordinated movement. Cross-crawls are really just the crawling pattern done while standing.

There are many different ways to perform the cross crawl. This is great, because we all have many different bodies and abilities. You can choose the cross crawl that is right for you based on your ability to perform it. This is one of the factors that makes cross crawls so effective. Anyone can do them, and they are easy to progress.

Cross-crawls can be performed in a chair, on the floor while lying on your back, while standing, walking, or even while skipping. If you cannot touch your opposite elbow to your opposite knee, you simply touch your opposite hand or forearm to your opposite knee or thigh. If you do not have the balance to perform the cross-crawl while standing, try it lying down on your back and do cross-crawl sit-ups. No matter what your abilities or physical limitations, you should be able to find a way to perform a cross-crawl.

Cross-crawls can easily be progressed to more challenging versions. For instance, if you have no trouble touching your elbow to your knee while standing, try doing them while you keep your fingertips behind your ears. If keeping your fingertips behind your ears is easy, try doing that with your eyes closed or with your eyes looking in the opposite direction of where you are rotating towards. Try cross-crawling marching forward, try cross-crawling while marching backwards, try them super slow, try them while skipping or even while skipping *and* spinning around in circles. You can even try them while eating green eggs and ham! Just kidding! Anyway, the more you can progress with your cross-crawls, the more coordination you are developing. However, you don't have to get fancy with your cross-crawls if you don't want to, they will still work. But, if you want to get as much out of them as you can, have fun and progress them. Just make sure you do them!

How to Roll

Rolling is simply the act of lying on the floor and transitioning from your belly to your back and from your back to your belly. There are more ways to roll than there are letters in the alphabet. But, for now, and because it works wonders in restoring movement patterns, we will roll the way Gray Cook outlines in his book *Movement*.

The following section on rolling comes from *Movement, pages 187 - 189* [35]*:*

Back to Belly Rolling - Upper Body

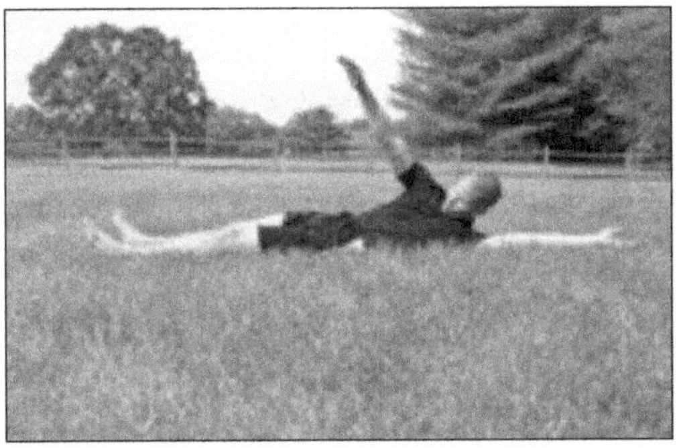

Lie on your back with your legs straight and your arms straight over head. Using your head, neck and right arm, reach across your body as far as you can and roll to your belly. Do not cheat and use your legs! Can you do this with both arms?

Belly to Back Rolling - Upper Body

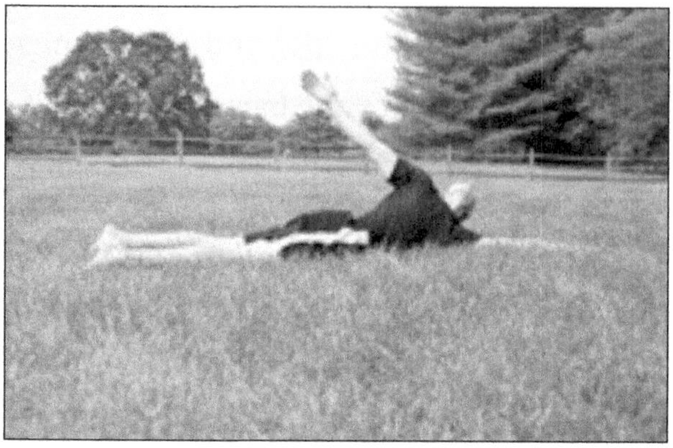

Lying on your belly with your legs straight and your arms straight over head, use your head, neck and right arm to reach back across your body and roll to your back. Do not cheat and use your legs! Can you do this with both arms?

Tip: Ever hear that the body will go where the head goes? We are wired that way. Use your eyes, neck and head to lead to where you want to roll. **You are training your vestibular system and your core muscles!**

And, it makes rolling so much easier!

Back to Belly Rolling - Lower Body

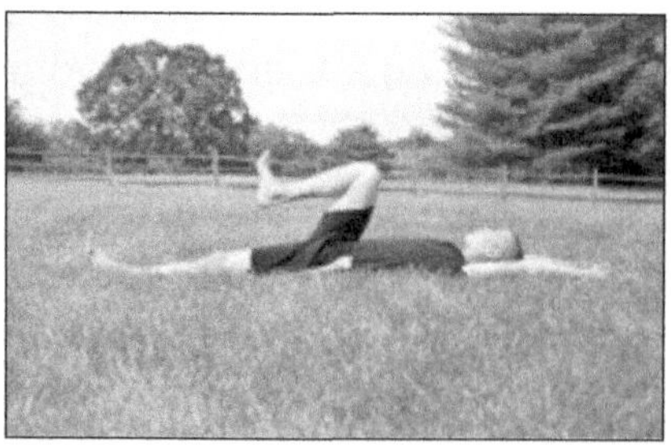

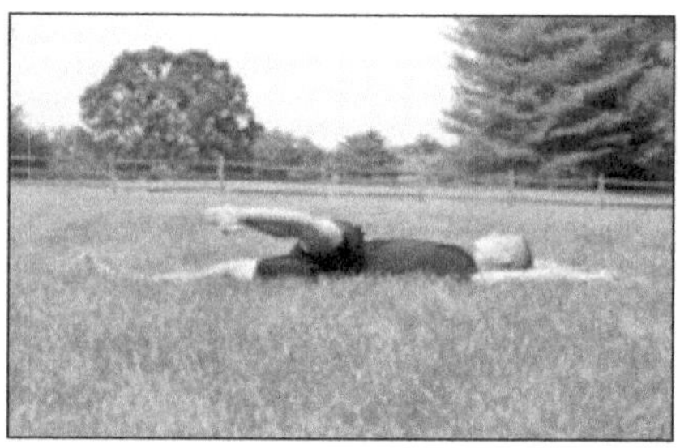

Lie on your back with your legs straight and your arms straight over head. Using your right leg, reach across your body and roll to your belly. Do not cheat and use your arms! Can you do this with both legs?

Belly to Back Rolling - Lower Body

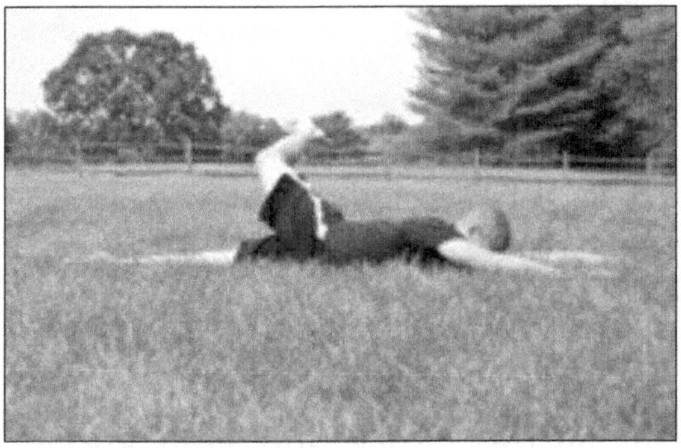

Lying on your belly with your legs straight and your arms straight over head, use your right leg to reach back across your body and roll to your back. Do not cheat and use your arms! Can you do this with both legs?

Tim likes to have his clients roll 3 times from each limb, in both directions. If a client has a hard time rolling, we know what we need to work on. He typically gives rolling as "homework." He likes for his clients to be able to fluidly roll from one side to the other with all their limbs with the same ease. Once this is accomplished, he starts introducing other forms of rolling; like only using the head and neck to roll, much like some babies do.

Again, there are several ways to roll. We like to use this method to start because it can expose movement issues and it works wonders for the client. We have witnessed rolling "fix", or clean up an entire Functional Movement Screen Score[36] in several of our clients. Rolling is how we start to learn and "earn" our movements and movement patterns as infants. It can also be a great way to re-learn and re-earn them again. Roll on, brother!

How to Rock

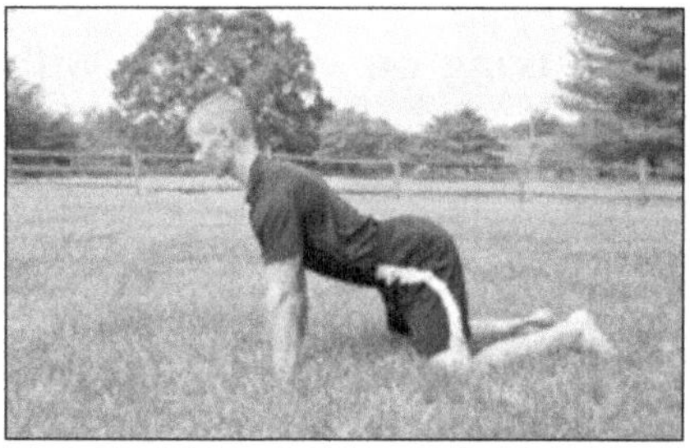

Starting Position

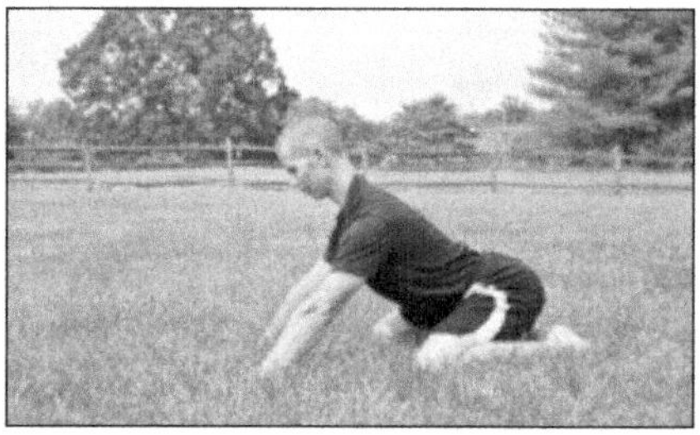

Ending Position

After the roll, you've got the rock. Rock and Roll! Rocking seems to be a great "reset" for a lot of people. Rocking is getting on your hands and knees, keeping a tall chest, or a long spine, and rocking your butt back towards your calves. With our clients, we have found that rocking really seems to help improve posture, reflexive stability, and mobility.

There are two ways to rock. One way, Gray Cook's way, is to compress a swiss ball between your butt and a wall.[37] As you compress the ball you want to keep a long spine or a tall chest. This keeps your spine from rounding. It may help to place a water bottle or rolled up towel on your lower back. If the bottle rolls off, you are not keeping a long spine. This is a fantastic drill and it yields many benefits. This drill can really help get a person "connected." By pushing a Swiss ball between your butt and a wall, you really get your inner core muscles and your pelvic floor muscles to fire. You are basically turning on your 3DX, or your "muscle girdle." This drill can really help with core and trunk stability. Good things happen when you get the pelvic floor to fire. As Dr. Theresa Nesbit likes to say, "There is no core without the floor."

The other way we like to rock is to simply get on your hands and knees, keep a longs spine, point the crown of your head to the sky and rock your butt back towards your calves. Simply rock back and forth, nice and slow. You can take your knees farther apart as your hips loosen up. This is a great drill for improving hip mobility, and it helps restore good posture. If you want to see how your muscles are wired to your neck, do some head nods while you are sitting back towards your calves. You will feel your whole back musculature "turn on." If you try to look over your shoulders to see your own butt, you will even feel the muscles around your scapula sink the scapula down towards your butt. Head position facilitates muscle actions / contractions. Play with it a little and you will see what we mean.

Rocking is a great drill. It helps with scapula stabilization, proprioception, posture, and hip mobility. It's also an effective drill to do between sets of squats, deadlifts, or kettlebell swings. It really seems to "clean up" movement.

How to Crawl

Remember, all the things that make cross-crawls so wonderful will also apply to crawling. Crawling, however, may offer even more benefits because it gets the mechanoreceptors in your palms involved, and it forces your shoulders and hips to work together. It also helps with scapular stability and thoracic mobility. Crawling is an easy way to start building a strong center. Now, let's learn how to crawl! I know what you're thinking: "Crawling? This is so simple, even a baby can do it." And, you're absolutely right. A baby can do it, but you, however, may not be able to do it quite so well. It turns out that a lifetime of not crawling with tons of sitting and no running can make crawling quite frustrating for adults. There are some of you reading this right now who cannot crawl well. Others of you may find that you can crawl forward well, but you can't crawl backwards to save your life. Crawling is not necessarily easy, but once you master it on your hands and knees, and then in the Spider-Man position, you are on your way to becoming bulletproof. Remember, if you are not crawling well, you are probably not walking and running well either!

To begin crawling, Start on your hands and knees with your head held up so you can see where you are going. "Head held up" simply means crown of your head to the sky, and does not mean hyperextend your neck. If you have neck discomfort while crawling, simply lower your head a bit and try to keep your eyes up. The crawling movement should be like cross-crawls; opposite limbs move together. That is your opposite arm and leg should be moving forward together when you start traversing the floor. If they are not, this is something you need to work on. If you can crawl forward easily, check to see if you can crawl backwards easily as well. If you cannot, you have found another area to focus on.

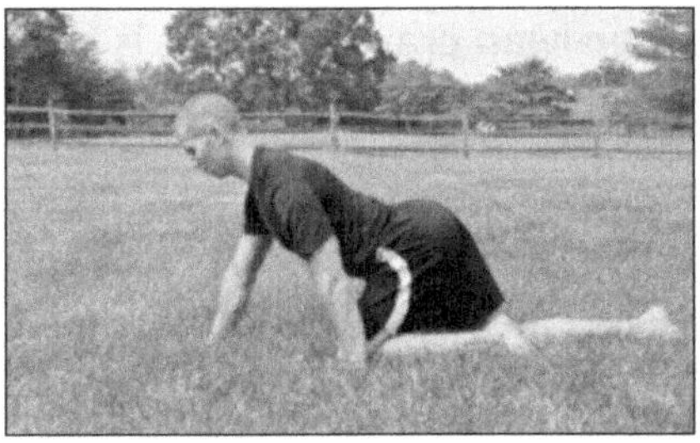

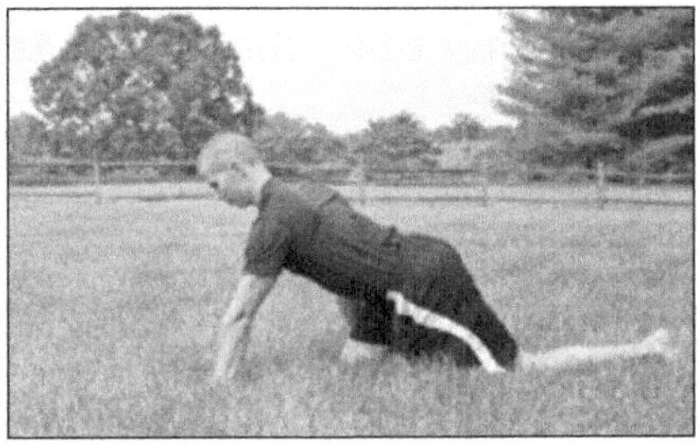

One of our favorite ways to crawl is the Spider-Man crawl, or the "Ninja" crawl. If you've ever seen a Spider-Man comic or cartoon, you know what we mean; your butt is kept low and your feet travel to the outsides of your arm. It is as if you are trying to sneak up on someone. We like this crawl because it gets the feet involved (more so if you are barefooted). Remember, your palms and feet are tied to your core musculature! Crawling is a great way to build reflexive stability!

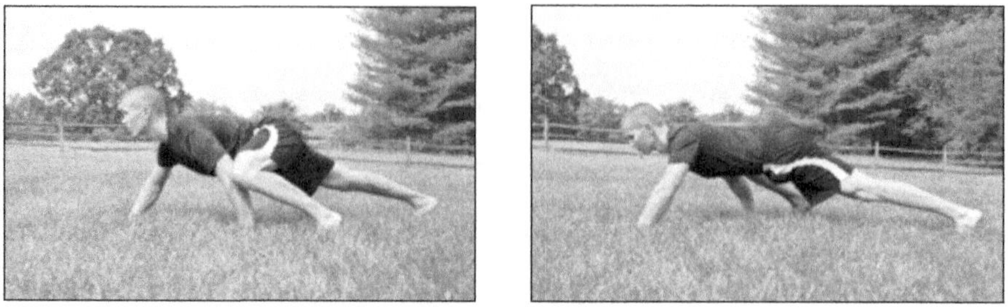

Spider-Man Crawl

Another thing that makes the Spider-Man crawl so great is that it is pretty much like "climbing" across the ground. Climbing is one of the best things we can do to build a fully capable body. Climbing is great for "tying the body together." Sadly though, most of us don't climb. The Spider-Man crawl is much like horizontal climbing. If you ever decide to take up climbing, this crawl can be a great way to get you prepared.

There are other ways to crawl, but we really like the "baby" crawl and the Spider-Man crawl. They have really worked well for us and our clients. The important thing is to crawl often because crawls, just like cross-crawls, can help your nervous system communicate better, and that can help you move better. Crawls can play a pivotal role in becoming bulletproof. Who cares how silly they make you look!

Using Your Breath to Press "Reset"

Breathing is also vital to becoming bulletproof. Everyone knows we need to breathe to live. No news there. But most of us are breathing wrong! When you are born, you are pretty much perfect from the start. You get some very primitive reflexes that are hard wired into you and from those, you get to build a whole host of movement patterns and abilities. Breathing is one reflex you are born with. It is also a reflex that you are capable of changing, or altering.

When you are born, you are a diaphragmatic breather. Or, a belly breather. Watch a new born baby, or an infant. Their little bellies go up and down when they breathe. They are taking full advantage of their lung volume by effortlessly breathing with their diaphragm (let's call that our "breathing muscle"). The diaphragm pulls a vacuum in the lungs allowing them to fill themselves full of life-giving air. The diaphragm, also massages the internal organs thus aiding in digestion. And, the diaphragm works with the pelvic floor to help create a reflexively stable core. Again, this is how we are born breathing - with our diaphragm.

Some of us, or most of us, end up retraining how we breathe by using our accessory muscles, or the muscles in our rib cage, neck and shoulders. These are the muscles a baby uses to breathe when his breathing is compromised and he is in distress. When babies use these muscles to breathe, they are usually sick and may need emergency medical attention. It may help to think of these as emergency breathing muscles. For some reason, whether it is due to our stressful lives, or because we are trying to hide our gut, we become "chest breathers," and we start using our accessory muscles to breathe.

Remember, the accessory breathing muscles are our "emergency" breathing muscles. We really don't need to be using these all the time. They are our startle, or fight or flight, muscles. Constantly breathing with our emergency muscles can cause a forward head carriage, neck pain, poor thoracic mobility, hunched forward posture, early fatigue when exercising, poor digestion, maybe even loss of our reflexive stability in our core muscles. If we are always breathing with our accessory muscles, our bodies are always in stress mode, which is a very inefficient, unhealthy mode to be stuck in for a long period of time. Some people spend a lifetime breathing like this.

The good news is if we can change our breathing pattern for the bad, then we can also retrain our breathing pattern for the good. Breathing is a natural reflex that is subconscious, however, breathing can also be controlled and trained consciously. Learning how to breath properly can unlock a whole host of health benefits and really put you on your way to becoming bulletproof.

From Tim

So how do we train ourselves to breathe using our diaphragm? I like the way Gray Cook and Brett Jones have been doing it; they use crocodile breathing.[38] In crocodile breathing, you lay on your belly and rest your forehead on the back of your hands. While inhaling through your nose, you want to try to breathe deep down into your belly. If you do this correctly, your belly will push against the floor and cause your lower back to rise up. The sides of your belly will also get wider, just like a crocodile! This is a very effective way to retrain yourself how to become a belly breather. At least it has worked well for me. Just 5 minutes a day can really go a long way towards reseting your proper breathing pattern.

Being a belly breather can go a long way towards becoming bulletproof. If you train with weights or if you lift heavy objects, using your diaphragm when you breathe allows you to create more inter-abdominal pressure.[39] That is to say, you can brace your body better to pick up a heavy load. It is kind of like zipping up a girdle around your midsection. Not only is this good for you, it could save you from a career ending injury!

Athletically speaking, being a belly breather will allow you to be more efficient in your day to day activities, as well as your sport of choice. This is because you are able to take in more air, and you are not using as much energy by breathing with your accessory muscles. Muscles require energy to contract. Constantly using your accessory muscles to breathe has a metabolic cost; you tire more quickly.

Being a belly breather may be one way to keep and/or regain a reflexively stable core. This is very important in day to day life because as we discussed earlier when talking about the 3D X, a reflexively stable core transfers forces from the ground through the torso efficiently. In other words, a reflexively stable core is crucial to becoming bulletproof because it yields a strong and stable body. If you do not have a reflexively strong center, your body will not be strong, and you will be more likely to get injured. Breathing, something you cannot live without doing, can be one of the best exercises you could engage in when it comes to becoming bulletproof.

From Mike:

My main message to take away from this section on breathing is to let it come naturally. Don't force anything. If you're crawling and rolling regularly and properly, diaphragmatic breathing comes naturally and becomes a necessity. Put your focus on eliminating tension as you crawl and roll and allow your body to naturally reset itself. If you spend too much time trying to get your breathing right, you'll find that you're going to generate the same unwanted and unnecessary tension that you get while you're on the phone, in traffic, or other stress-induced situations.

Reset your Feet!

If everything about your body is integrated, it would make sense that becoming bulletproof requires a multi-faceted approach. Having said that, your feet play no small part when it comes to building a resilient body. Believe it or not, we are born without shoes. Yes, it is true. When you came into the world, your feet were bare. They were perfectly made to grasp the ground and give you a platform on which to stand. Feet, much like the hands, are full of nerve endings that send proprioceptive information to your brain. In other words, the nerves in your feet help paint a picture in your brain of where your body is and what it is doing.

When you learned to crawl, or traverse the floor, your feet sent all kinds of information to your brain about what your body was doing. Your feet sent information to your leg muscles and your core muscles as well and they helped establish some of your movement patterns. Remember, everything about you is tied together. Nothing is isolated. Your feet have sensory nerves and proprioceptors to help complete the "body map" in your brain.

Remember the analogy of the 3D map of your body inside your brain? The more clear the map is, the better you move. If the map is fuzzy, you may not move so well. If you are getting good information from all your sensory nerves in your skin, joints and muscles, your movement map will be clearer. If you are not getting good information from your sensory nerves, your movement map will get fuzzy.

Shoes can make your movement map fuzzy because they prevent your feet from feeling the world. Shoes do not allow your feet to feel the ground. Shoes do not allow your feet to move as they were designed to move. Shoes do not allow your foot muscles to work the way they were designed. There are nerves in our skin, muscles and joints that all help paint the picture of our movement map. A shoe effectively distorts all of these!

A foot has joints. It is made to bear weight and move. A foot also has muscles to support those joints and to support our entire structure. A foot obviously has skin to protect us, as well as give our brain feedback for the environment we are in. Shoes can compress the feet, not allowing the muscles to function or the joints to move. This distorts the proprioceptive information being received by the brain. It also weakens the muscles in the foot. (Use it or lose it!) This can cause us to become flat-footed because we lose our arches, those wonderfully strong structures that are made to withstand huge amounts of compressive force.[40] Shoes also distort the sensory information being given by the skin.

If our goal is to become as resilient as possible, it may be a good idea to spend some time barefooted, especially when you train. Remember, everything about you is connected. All of our proprioceptive information gets routed through our vestibular system first, *and* our vestibular system is connected to our core musculature. It would only be a small leap of faith to think that your feet are connected to your core as well. The truth is they are! Pavel Tsatsouline points out, "...Another power boosting reflex is called the positive support reaction. This reflex causes the leg musculature to contract in response to the pressure on the sole of the foot."[41] Pavel also goes on to mention the *extensor reflex* which causes the leg muscles to fire in a precise pattern depending on how the foot hits the ground.[42] The leg muscles are indeed part of the core, and they certainly would affect how forces travel from the ground through the core. You want your leg muscles prepared for the forces you are about to absorb and produce from the ground. In other words, your feet are important! They prepare the body for power, stability and strength. Shoes only distort, alter and slow information from the feet to the brain.

Again, going barefoot may be the way to go if you're trying to become bulletproof. I'm not saying you can never wear shoes, but I would suggest when you train, or play, you allow your feet to feel the ground. If the idea of being barefoot gives you the willies, you can always try barefoot shoes, or minimalist shoes. They will allow your foot to perform as it was designed. There are several new minimalist shoe options available now that the barefoot movement is catching on.

If you haven't spent anytime being barefoot since you were a toddler and you decide to give being barefoot a try, use common sense. Ease your way into it. Remember, becoming bulletproof is a journey, not a one time event. Your body and your feet will be grateful if you make this transition gradually. It is no different than beginning an exercise program, you ease your way into it to become successful.

From Tim:

I would like to add that crawling around like Spiderman while you are barefooted is a great way to ease your foot into barefoot training. When you are in the Spiderman position, you have considerably reduced the load on your feet. In other words, your feet get to "strength train" with only a fraction of your weight. Yet another benefit to crawling!

Engaging Everyday

All right, here is where we lay out the method for becoming bulletproof. These "reset" drills, or exercises, can be done anytime or several times throughout the day. But let's face it, people like structure. So, we'll try to give you a little structure here so that you can sleep peacefully at night.

The best time to perform the "reset button" drills is right before you train. You can use them as a warm-up. There are many, many fitness experts out there right now who don't believe we should have to "warm up." They say we should just be able to engage in our chosen exercise. Well, they are right. We should be able to simply engage in our chosen exercise session or event. But the truth is, we just don't do a lot of things we should be able to do in the first place. For instance, we should be able to stand for hours on end, not sit. We should be able to run for miles without tiring. We simply don't move and use our bodies the way they were intended to be used. So, until we do start living the way we were designed, it may be a wise idea to "warm-up" a little before we train.

The time right before your training session is a great time to perform the midline crossing, or cross-lateral movements. At most, it will take 5 minutes out of your day. Some people will need to perform certain midline crossing drills, while others may not. For example, if you cannot roll from your back to your belly using your legs or arms independently, you should probably focus on that a little. Or, if you cannot crawl like Spider-Man, you should probably spend more time crawling on your hands and knees until you can.

Though we have not found any solid sequence to performing any of these drills, it would make sense from a child development perspective that there would be a logical order. However, not all babies develop the same. Some skip steps, some crawl backwards, some don't crawl at all, though they probably should! The same goes for adults. You need what *you need*. You may need to do a ton of crawling, but not so much rolling. Or you may need a lot of rolling and not so much crawling. We don't know what you need, but we do know it won't hurt you to do them all! That way, you get what you need. Again, we don't think the order matters as much as getting the reps in, so you don't always have to do everything in the same order every single day. You can go "crazy" and mix it up a bit if you like! Having said all of that, we start almost everyone out with cross-crawls. Everyone can do those regardless of their abilities.

If there is any "magic ingredient" to anything we are about to share with you, it is simply this: consistency. Consistency is the only thing that works and it is the only thing that will guarantee your success. If we did provide for you the perfect way to train, the best method ever, it would not matter one single bit if you did not apply the information consistently. ***If it is important, do it everyday...***[43] By the way, it is important!

On days you are training or *playing*, we recommend the following:

Preset Yourself and Press "Reset" (Warm up):

Cross crawls, 20 times

Roll, 3 times each way

Rock, 5 to 10 times

Crawl, 20 steps forward (baby-style until you own Spider-Man style and forward until you own backwards)

Once you have pressed reset, you are ready to move, or play, or train. It doesn't matter what you call it as long as you do it. So, insert your favorite activity here.

"Reset" yourself again (Cool down):

Cross crawls, 20 times

Crawl, 20 steps forward

On days you are not training, spend some time **playing** in and with these movements. Do cross-crawls super slow (huge benefit to this!).[44] Do them with your eyes closed (be careful). Do them with your finger tips behind your ears if you have the mobility. Do them while you walk. Do them while you skip. Explore the movement and be creative. There are huge benefits in all of this.

Learn to roll in different ways. Think of as many ways to roll as you can. Learn how to use your neck to roll (this is huge!!!). Learn to perform Gray Cook's "Hard Roll"; it's really hard. To learn the Hard Roll, check out Gray Cook's DVD, *The Secrets of Primitive Patterns.*

Practice rocking into a stability ball. Practice rocking with your eyes closed. Practice raising your head while you rock. We have even found some very weird effects if you practice rocking while you are visualizing, or staring at, the center of an X. We have used this to quiet pain in ourselves and our friends with great success.

When crawling, can you crawl backwards as well as you can crawl forward? If not, learn to crawl backward. It will pay off huge returns in your coordination, among many other benefits. Practice crawling like Spider-Man or a ninja. Be slow, be quiet, be creative!

Have fun. Yes, this seems silly! But you know what? It can help you regain the body you were meant to have.

Choose to engage and move every day. Movement is the key to becoming bulletproof. It is the key to life. The next few chapters are intended to help you structure a movement plan and build a solid foundation on which to achieve a resilient, healthy body.

Go Outside and Play!

We can learn a lot from watching children and even more from acting like them. This is perhaps the most important concept of this book. Whether or not you believe rolling around on the floor and crawling around like Spider-Man are the miracle reset for your body, you must learn how to play. We were simply made to be able to move, and we just don't do what we were designed to do. That is the bottom line.

Do you remember how good you always felt and how much energy you always had as a child? Ever notice how resilient kids are? Do you think we start slowing down and getting injured because we grow old? Or, do you think maybe we grow old and start slowing down because we stop playing? That is definitely something worth pondering.

We need to relearn how to play! Ask any kid what his or her favorite part of school is, and he or she will tell you it is recess, the part of the day when they get to go outside and play. That is, of course, at schools where recess is still allowed! We as adults need to learn how to go outside and play. Play can be anything you enjoy doing. It can be a game of basketball, riding a bike, going out for a run, climbing a tree, or anything else you enjoy doing that gets you moving. It doesn't matter what activity you chose for your play day, just DO SOMETHING! It can be almost anything as long as you do it. The more fun the better. Just 15 to 30 minutes, it doesn't matter. Just do something - consistently (that is the key).

Seriously, go find a playground at a local park, and be a kid! You will be amazed at how good you start to feel. Why? Because you will start using your body the way it was intended. You will start feeling good. You will not only be exercising your body, but also your brain. Maybe you'll relearn some movement patterns, cement some new neural connections in your brain, release some positive hormones in your body, reduce your stress, improve your energy, learn to laugh, etc. The list of benefits just goes on and on.

From Tim:

Learning how to play is crucial for becoming bulletproof. Set aside 2 to 3 days a week to be creative and have fun for 15 to 30 minutes. For my play, I like to crawl around while pretending to be Spider-Man. Sometimes I like to run sprints or climb trees. The key is I'm having fun, and I'm doing something. Mike likes to play with agility drills, kettlebells and bodyweight exercises. Again, he is having fun and he is doing something.

To most of you reading this, our chosen activities of play will not seem much like play at all! That is okay. Play can be anything, it doesn't really matter what you choose. What matters is that you engage, have fun, and make play a regular part of your life.

I know this will be a challenge for most of you reading this. You have the freedom to be creative and design your own play dates. You can use your own creativity and do whatever you like. If you are really de-conditioned, start out gradually. Maybe set aside ten to fifteen minutes to get outside and play a few times a week. As you start feeling better and more conditioned, increase your time and/or your level of activity. The bottom line is do something, move, and have fun. It really is that simple.

In case it helps to get your creative juices flowing, here are some examples of play:

1. Play dodge-ball with your kids.
2. Go for a walk, or a run, in a park.
3. Go bike riding with some friends. Wear your helmet!
4. Play tennis.
5. Learn how to run sprints.
6. Climb a tree or play on some monkey bars.
7. Learn to swim.
8. Play frisbee.
9. Wii yoga!
10. Sign up for a 5k and raise money for a charity.

Playing may surprise you. You may find that you start enjoying it. You may even find yourself doing things you never thought you would do like signing up for a 5k or joining group bicycle rides. Engaging in play and being active can lead to all sorts of new activities and hobbies. Learning how to play can lead you to a whole new lifestyle. Play can lead to living!

If you would like a more structured plan for play, or a more advanced plan, Mike has designed several small "play sessions" to get you started. Some of the following "play sessions" may be seen as full blown workouts. To some people, that is play. Remember, *these are just examples!* Choose the ones you would like to do. Leave the ones you would not want to do. Adjust, change, and tinker with them as you like.

From Mike:

The important thing is to do something that gets you moving every day. Modern humans are creatures of habit, but think back to our ancestors. Every day was a new and novel stimulus. From day to day you never knew whether you would be running from predators, hunting game, migrating, etc. So in order to capitalize on our need for fresh stimulus, our "play dates" should encompass a wide variety of movement. The following are just examples. Feel free to add your own, just remember to have FUN!

1. Every minute on the minute alternate between 5 pull-ups and 10 bodyweight squats. Do this for 20 minutes.
2. Run backwards for 100 steps, drop and do 10 pushups. Side shuffle for 100 steps, drop and do 10 pushups. Skip for 100 steps, drop and do 10 pushups. Run high knees for 100 steps, drop and do 10 pushups. Sprint for 100 steps, drop and do 10 pushups. Repeat as many times as you can in 20 minutes.
3. Find a hill. Sprint up the hill and Spider-Man crawl back down. Repeat five times.
4. Complete the following for time: Do 1 pushup, then 1 burpee. Then 2 pushups, then 2 burpees. Complete that to 10 reps, then start descending back down to 1.
5. Mark off 100 yards. Do as many broad jumps as necessary to reach the end.
6. Do 25 kettlebell swings, then 25 pushups. Then 20 kettlebell swings, then 20 pushups. 15 kettlebell swings, 15 pushups. 10 kettlebell swings, 10 pushups. 5 kettlebell swings, 5 pushups. Complete as many rounds as possible in 20 minutes.
7. Alternate between pull-ups and pushup ladders. Do one pull-up, then one pushup. Add a rep until you can't complete in good form. Then start over at one. Complete as many rounds as possible in 10 minutes.

8. 50 kettlebell swings, then sprint 50 yards. Walk back. Complete 5 times.
9. Sprint 10 yards, jog back. Sprint 20 yards, jog back. Sprint 30 yards, jog back. Sprint 40 yards, jog back. Sprint 50 yards, jog back. Complete twice.
10. Skip rope for 20 UNBROKEN jumps, then 10 pushups. Add 20 jumps and 10 pushups each round. Complete this until you have 100 jumps and 50 pushups.
11. Spider-Man crawl for 100 yards.
12. Summersault 10 times, baby crawl 10 yards, Spider-Man crawl 10 yards, sprint 10 yards, broad jump 10 yards. Complete as many times as you can in 20 minutes.
13. Reverse lunge 15 steps per leg, do 10 pushups, then sprint back to starting point. Repeat 5 times.
14. Do 5 pull-ups or chin-ups, then 10 sit-ups. Keep going until you have done 25 pull/ chin ups and 50 sit-ups.
15. Jog a mile.
16. Skip a mile.
17. Skip 100 yards, then backwards run to the start. Do continuously for 10 minutes.
18. Do 5 pushups, then 1 broad jump. 10 pushups, then 1 broad jump. 15 Pushups, then 1 broad jump. 20 pushups, then 1 broad jump. 25 pushups, then 1 broad jump. Complete twice.

19. Do 5 sit ups, then 5 rolls. 5 sit ups, then roll back to start. Do this continuously for 10 minutes.
20. Walk or jog 100 yards, then do 10 pushups. Repeat until you have done 100 pushups.

Strength Training

From Tim:

Strength training can also play a pivotal role in becoming bulletproof. I don't know of anyone who could not benefit from getting stronger. Having strength is like having armor. It can protect you from unfortunate injuries, and it can enable you to perform unusual tasks. Strength makes you resilient.

In 1989, Dr. Phillip Maffetone wrote a book called *In Fitness and In Health: Everyone is an Athlete.* I love this concept. I love it because deep down, I know it is true. Think about it. You are an athlete. You were made to move. You were perfectly designed in every way.

We are all athletes. Therefore, we should all train like athletes. A professional athlete usually strength trains no more than twice a week during the season of their sport. The rest of their week, they practice their sport and their skills and then they play their sport. One day when I was talking to Mike about our ideas on training, he said one of the most brilliant things I have ever heard. "You should train the way an elite athlete trains for their sport. Your sport is life." That is an awesome statement! Our sport is life and we should be prepared for it.

Here is our training plan to prepare you for the "Sport of Life" and whatever it throws at you:

Strength train twice a week. Then, PLAY (do something) the rest of the week. Earth shattering we know. But, it works. It works for elite athletes, and it will work for you. Best of all, it is SIMPLE.

If you are new to the idea of strength training, it may be a good idea to start strength training by learning how to move your own body and use your own bodyweight. You can develop really good levels of strength and a great physique just by learning how to use your own body.

Remember the lowly pushup? It is a tremendous whole body strength developer! A perfect pushup requires strength! Is a perfect pushup too challenging for you? Start Spider-Man crawling! You will develop the strength you need to perform the pushup. Yes, even crawling can be strength training.

If you are a beginner, I think it is a really good idea to learn how to do a few basic moves to help you get started.

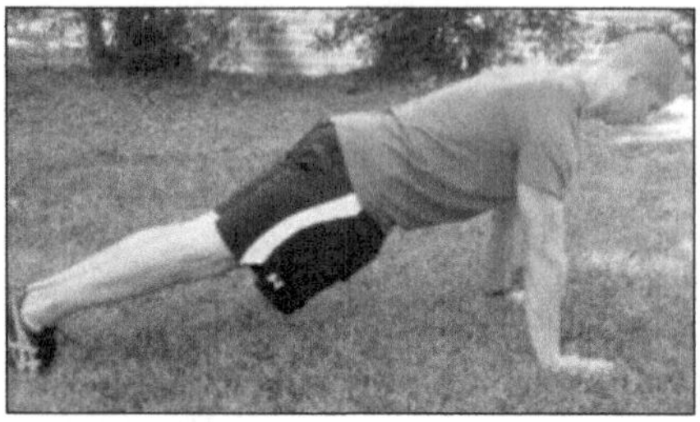

The mighty pushup!

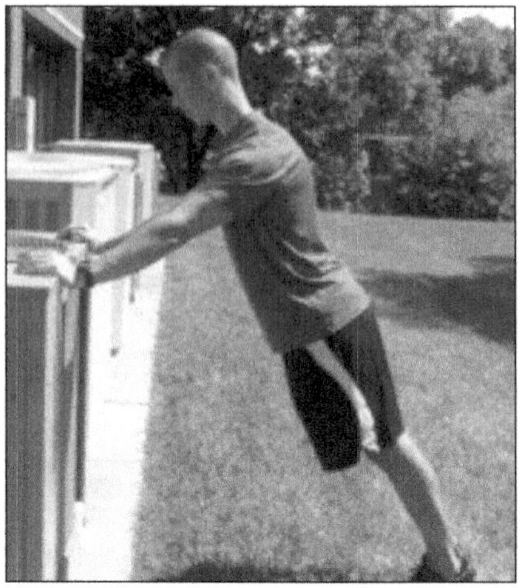

The incline pushup

- Learn how to do a pushup. If you can't do one on the floor, learn how to do them from an incline position or from your knees.
- Learn how to squat. Squatting is a pattern you once had as a child, and it is a pattern you need to keep.

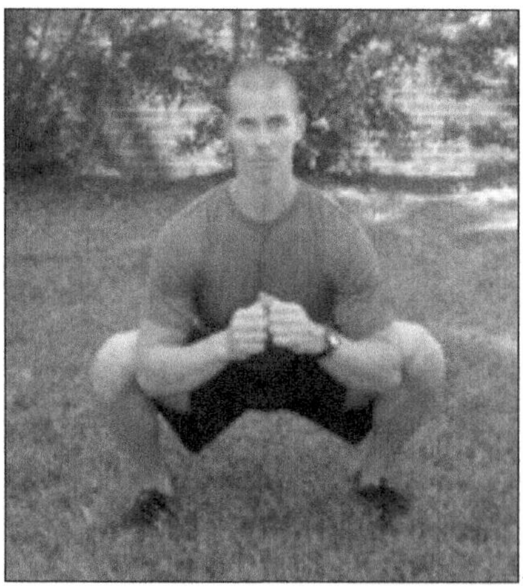

The bodyweight squat

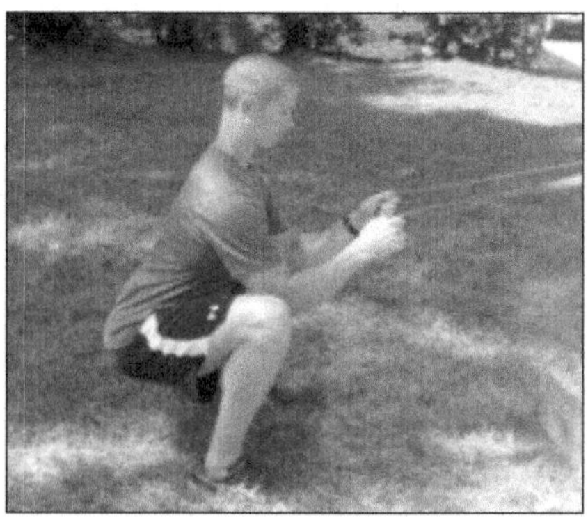

The assisted squat using a strap

The following program is a *simple* strength training program for **beginners**. It can be done by almost anyone, and it will get you stronger and ready for more challenging exercises:

First, pick two days a week to strength train, like maybe Monday and Thursday or

Tuesday and Saturday. Just pick two days with ample recovery time in between them.

Days 1 and 2:

Warm-up by pressing reset.

Perform 5 perfect pushups for 5 sets

Perform 10 bodyweight squats for 5 sets

Spider-man crawl for 3 minutes - if you have to rest, rest. But try for a total crawl-time of

3 minutes.

Each week, try to add another set to your pushups and squats until you are able to perform 20 sets of 5 pushups and 10 sets of 10 squats for a total of 100 each. Also, once you can perform the spider-man crawl for a continuous 3 minutes, start adding 30 seconds of crawl-time each week until you can crawl for 5 minutes.

Once you have accomplished this, it is time to change it up just a little:

Days 1 and 2:

Warm-up by pressing reset.

Perform 10 perfect pushups for 5 sets

Perform 20 bodyweight squats for 5 sets

Spider-man crawl backwards for 3 minutes - if you have to rest, rest. But try for a total crawl-time of 3 minutes.

Each week, try to add another set to your pushups and squats until you are able to perform 10 sets of 10 pushups and 10 sets of 20 squats. Also, once you can perform the backwards Spider-Man crawl for a continuous 3 minutes, start adding 30 seconds of crawl-time each week until you can crawl for 5 minutes.

Once you have accomplished this, congratulations! You are stronger and you are now ready to explore more levels of strength training, like maybe Mike's following plan for more seasoned weightlifters.

From Mike:

As Tim discussed earlier, we believe that life is a sport and all of us are participating athletes. Therefore we should look at how in season athletes train. The vast majority strength train two days a week with the bulk of their time and energy being devoted to their sport specific skill work. We need to remember that an athletes time in the weight room is nothing more than GPP (general physical preparedness) for us. Your sport isn't lifting weights.

Lifting weights is just a tool to enhance the other activities you participate in.

We recommend two days of strength training per week, with anywhere between three to five days of "play" or sport specific skill work. It is my opinion that the bulk of your strength work should be broken down into the four major lifts: Squat, Overhead Press, Deadlift and Bench Press. Combine that with bodyweight work, sprints and other forms of play and you should be on your way to becoming bulletproof.

The following template has proved very successful for me and my clients in the past:

Week One

Day 1

1A) Overhead Press:
5 reps at 65%
5 reps at 75%
5 reps at 85%
10 reps at 65%

1B) Pullups (varying grips):
5 sets of 3-5 reps

2A) Deadlifts (Trap Bar or Conventional):
5 reps at 65%
5 reps at 75%
5 reps at 85%
10 reps at 65%

2B) Dips: 5 sets of 10-15 reps

3) Cross Body Sit Ups (on a slant board if available): 3 sets of 10 reps

Free Time: 10 minutes to do whatever you want (curls, flyes, etc). The important point to remember is that whatever you do should enhance your main lifts, not detract from them.

Day 2

1A) Bench Press:

5 reps at 65%

5 reps at 75%

5 reps at 85%

10 reps at 65%

1B) Pullups (varying grips):

5 sets of 3-5 reps

2A) Squats:

5 reps at 65%

5 reps at 75%

5 reps at 85%

10 reps at 65%

2B) Dips:

5 sets of 10-15 reps

3) Situps: 3 sets of 10 reps

Free Time: Same as above

Week 2

Day 1

1A) Overhead Press:

3 reps at 70%

3 reps at 80%

3 reps at 90%

10 reps at 70%

1B) Pullups (varying grips):

5 sets of 3-5 reps

2A) Deadlifts:

3 reps at 70%

3 reps at 80%

3 reps at 90%

10 reps at 70%

2B) Dips:

5 sets of 10-15 reps

3) Situps: 4 sets of 10 reps

Day 2

1A) Bench Press:

3 reps at 70%
3 reps at 80%
3 reps at 90%
10 reps at 70%

1B) Pullups:

5 sets of 3-5 reps

2A) Squats:

3 reps at 70%
3 reps at 80%
3 reps at 90%
10 reps at 70%

2B) Dips

5 sets of 10-15 reps

3) Situps:

4 sets of 10 reps

Free Time: Same as above

Week 3

Day 1

1A) Overhead Press:

5 reps at 75%
3 reps at 85%
3 reps at 95%
10 reps at 75%

1B) Pullups (varying grips):

5 sets of 3-5 reps

2A) Deadlifts (Trap Bar or Conventional):

5 reps at 75%
3 reps at 85%
3 reps at 95%
10 reps at 75%

2B) Dips:

5 sets of 10-15 reps

3) Cross Body Sit Ups (on a slant board if available): 5 sets of 10 reps

Free Time: Same as above.

Day 2

1A) Bench Press:

5 reps at 75%
3 reps at 85%
3 reps at 95%
10 reps at 75%

2A) Squats:

5 reps at 75%
3 reps at 85%
3 reps at 95%
10 reps at 75%

1B) Pullups (varying grips):

5 sets of 3-5 reps

2B) Dips:

5 sets of 10-15 reps

3) Situps:

5 sets of 10 reps

Free Time: Same as above.

Now, when choosing the weight that you will be basing your percentages off of, what we recommend is that you pick your max weight and then reduce it by 10-15%. This will be the "training max" that you base your training percentages off of. For instance, if your max weight is 100 lbs, your training weight would be 85 lbs. Now for some of you this may seem unbelievably light. Good. This will ensure perfect form and perpetual progress. In addition, you won't feel too burned out to take advantage of the "play dates". Remember as athletes our sport isn't lifting weights.

After each three week block I want you to add 5 lbs to your upper body max and 10 lbs to your lower body max then recalculate your percentages again. This will provide your training numbers for the next cycle.

It is always better to start off too light. If you pick a weight that is too heavy, you run the risk of over taxing your central nervous system or sacrificing form for weight.

Heads Up!

Since we were just discussing strength training, We thought this would be a good place to talk about *our opinion* on head position. There is a big debate in the training community regarding where your head should be while you are training or performing certain exercises. Really, it is a question of neck position, not so much head position, though you can't have one without the other.

Our position is this: go with nature. We are designed so that our heads stay up, on the horizon. For an overly simple example, our vestibular system is like a built in gyroscope inside your head, it is self-righting in that our heads naturally want to be up. It simply isn't natural for us to keep our head still or not move our neck while the rest of the body is moving.

Look at a baby as he is learning to crawl. A child's head is up, so he can see where he is going. This is one of the ways we develop our eyesight as well as hand-eye coordination. Remember also that our vestibular system is tied to our core. The old adage that where the head goes, the body will follow is true. The position of our head and neck can facilitate better flexion or extension from our core musculature. Want better extension? Keep your head up. Want better flexion? Keep your head down. Try it yourself. If you are familiar with yoga, perform an upward dog and then perform a downward dog a few times. Then try doing them again, but lead the motion with your head first. Do you notice how much easier and more "open" you feel when you lead with your head?

Again, our opinion differs with the popular notion of keeping a neutral neck (inline with the spine) when training. Yes, your neck may be "safe" if you can hold it neutral, but that does not mean it is a natural position. As Mike has said, "We have tried to outsmart what we were designed to do." We (the fitness community) place a lot of rules on the body when it comes to movement, yet none of us came with a movement manual when we were born! Maybe we should just look at how we were designed, perfectly designed, by the way. Imagine a short stop in his athletic ready stance with his neck held in a neutral position. How would he ever make a play? He can't see the ball, he can't react. Weight training is not baseball, I know. But it is an athletic event. It is movement. When in life do we move the body without allowing the neck to move? Why would we place this rule on the body when it comes to picking stuff up? If we weren't supposed to do it, why do we do it so well and so easily, so instinctively?

Don’t get us wrong, we are not talking about hyperextension of the neck. Too much of anything can be a bad thing. Right? We are talking about holding the crown of the head towards the sky; the head is held up like babies do when they crawl so the eyes are in place to see the world. Heads up! The way we were designed.

Nutrition Matters

From Mike:

Nutrition is one of the most highly debated topics in the field of diet and exercise. High carb, low carb, Paleo diets, high protein, high fat, low fat, Atkins, etc. The list goes on and on. The main thing all advocates can agree on is that there needs to be some sort of structure to your eating.

The most recent structure has been the very successful multiple meal plan. This is where an individual will consume anywhere from 4-6 small meals throughout the day. The idea behind this is to mimic the way a baby eats as he or she is growing. Supposedly this eating plan will stave off catabolism (muscle wasting) and prime your body for growth. It does work. I followed it myself for many years with good results. However, I started looking for better, i.e., easier ways to do things. I hated being a slave to the clock for eating. Do you know how annoying it is to your friends and family when you need to stop whatever you're doing every 2-3 hours to ingest a meal?

What I started realizing was that this system was another example of society trying to fit a square peg into a round hole. Babies eat this way because they are constantly synthesizing new tissue and growing at an incredible rate. The average adult is not. Babies also eat this way because they are hungry this often. The average adult is not. So, how do we reconcile these ideas? We examine the principles behind them. Namely, eat when you're hungry and eat for what you have done, not what you are going to do. Keep things as simple as possible.

Everyone says breakfast is the most important meal of the day, but how many times have you gotten up in the morning and not been hungry? Quite a few people don't start getting hungry until mid morning or early afternoon. And this makes sense, because when you first get up, you haven't done anything.

My system is very simple. It starts with a full 32 hour fast. Now this may seem like a long time but consider that for at least 16 of those 32 hours you will be asleep. You would start your fast on a Saturday night when you go to bed. Don't eat anything all day Sunday, then go to bed. On Monday, begin your day as normal but only eat as you get hungry and only eat for what you have done. In other words, there is no need for a big lumberjack breakfast when all you've done is get out of bed. If you start getting hungry mid-morning, then have a small snack; preferably something high in protein, like nuts or yogurt. Then, go about your day as usual. Enjoy you're workout, then when you're done with the exertion and you feel your appetite returning, dig in! It makes the most sense to consume the bulk of your calories in the evening before going to sleep because that is when your body will be attempting to repair itself. You want to give it the necessary materials to rebuild when the construction crew shows up!

My personal favorite way to enhance this protocol is to include 50-100g of PeptoPro® from True Protein (www. Trueprotein.com) mixed in throughout the day. I like to mix up the PeptoPro® in a gallon jug of Crystal Light® and drink it throughout the day. This serves multiple functions for me. One, it ensures I'm taking in enough water. Two, PeptoPro® is so quickly digested that it creates a very fast spike of aminos in my system but also leaves very quickly allowing me to get back to a fasting/fat burning state. Three, the PeptoPro® is extremely high in L-Leucine, which is the principle amino responsible for protein synthesis.

So, throughout the day I will just drink my PeptoPro®. Then, when it comes time for dinner, I will eat according to my hunger levels. I always take in a source of protein first, then eat whatever else I desire to fulfill my caloric requirements. This serves multiple functions for me as well. It allows me to have quite a bit of variety in my diet. It allows me to eat dinner with friends or family with little dietary restrictions because I can pretty much eat whatever I want while staying lean. I just have to stop when I'm full. In addition, eating this way creates a very nice caloric fluctuation from day to day, which ensures that my metabolism stays "flexible" rather than getting adapted to a constant source of calories.

From Tim:

Mike's above plan may seem a little drastic to some of you. All I can say is that Mike knows his stuff when it comes to nutrition. Both of us have been eating this way for a while, and it has allowed me to stay extremely lean. I have enjoyed good energy and strength eating this way, and I now enjoy eating "real food" in the evenings. Having said that, I know eating this way is not for everyone. So, here is my take on nutrition:

Nutrition is important. It is an integral part, or piece to the puzzle, when it comes to becoming bulletproof. You can't expect to become healthy if you eat Twinkies all the time!

I am not going to tell you how you should eat. I am going to tell you that it is your fault if you don't eat well. If you want to be bulletproof, you simply cannot eat Oreos everyday and wonder why you are not making any progress. Most of us are not vegetarians or meatetarians. We are junketarians.

Perhaps the biggest secret to eating well and maximizing your potential is simply taking responsibility for what you are putting in your mouth. For example, if you eat potato chips or cheesy poofs everyday, you are not a victim of your diet. You are the perpetrator! Oreos just don't jump down your mouth without your help.

We, as a society just don't take responsibility for our actions, especially when it comes to eating.

"I just can't seem to lose any weight." People say that all the time. Yet, they forget that they have been through the fast food drive-thru three times this week. Was there a tractor beam that pulled them into the drive-thru or did they simply choose to visit the fast food restaurant? *Most of the time*, it is our own eating habits and choices that determine how much we weigh, how we feel, and how we perform. You simply cannot expect to have great health and be bulletproof if you eat junk all the time. You must take responsibility for what you eat. You are not a victim.

There is a ton of great information out there when it comes to nutrition. You can learn about macro-nutrient ratios, the glycemic index, fiber, water intake and all kinds of eating plans. Do yourself a favor and learn about food. Hire a nutritionist. If you don't have the time and energy for that, simply eat natural, non-processed foods. If God made it, it's probably good for you. If man made it, it is probably junk. Learn how to shop, learn how to eat, learn how to make good decisions. If you want a way to hold yourself accountable, keep a food journal and record everything you eat and review it each night. Nutrition is not rocket science. You are completely capable or figuring this out. If you are serious about becoming healthy and resilient, you *must* figure this out!

Again, there is no magic eating plan. Any diet can work if it fits into your lifestyle and you can *consistently* apply it. If you want more direction and you simply want a specific plan to follow, research the following:

Precision Nutrition

The Paleo Diet

The Zone

The Warrior Diet

Weight Watchers

The Maker's Diet

Jack Lalanne used to have a saying, "Exercise is king, Nutrition is queen. Put them together and you have a happy kingdom." I'm going to miss Jack. He was THE visionary who put fitness on the map. Jack knew his stuff. Nutrition is queen when it comes to becoming bulletproof!

The Magic Bullet to Complete Physical Success

Is there a magic bullet to becoming bulletproof? Yes. Yes there is. There is one "magic" key to unlocking the body of your dreams. That key is simple consistency. I know this was already touched on earlier, but I believe this topic bears repeating.

Simple consistency is the key to unlocking almost any goal.

Think about it. What is the best way to prevent cavities? By taking care of your teeth. And how do you do that? You brush them 2 to 3 times every day. Every single day.

The best plans in the world for any goal or endeavor will fail if consistent application is not applied. The best "diet" will not work if you do not consistently apply its principles. The best workout regimen ever invented will never produce the results it promises if it is not applied daily. You hold the keys to unlocking your fitness goals, or any goal for that matter. You must consistently engage.

"If it is important, do it everyday." - Dan John, who credits Dan Gable, wrestling phenom and legend. Those words are worth etching in your head with a permanent marker. If you want to unlock your full potential, you must engage daily. Whether it is your relationship with your spouse you want to improve, whether you want to lose 30 lbs, or you just want less cavities when you go to the dentist for your routine teeth cleaning, you must engage daily in the activities that will yield your desired outcome(s).

Jack Lalanne is a hero of mine (Tim). Jack is pretty much the father of fitness in this country as we know it. He died this year at the age of 96 years old. At the age of 96, he had more energy, strength and stamina than most of today's 20-somethings do. He could still do finger tip pushups at 96 years old! How many of those can you do? You want to know what Jack's big secret was to his health and longevity? It was consistency. Every single day of his life, Jack exercised. Jack moved. Jack did something. He made a consistent effort to move his body everyday. And in his 90s he could still out work, out last and out perform most of this country's population. Jack knew the secret to a happy, healthy life. More than that, Jack took action and applied that secret to his **daily** life-style. Jack did something every day.

Conclusion

When we decided to write this book and present this information, our only motives were to learn how to become as resilient as possible and to help others do the same. This is important to us because we both believe that a healthy, strong body leads to a healthy, happy life.

There is a ton of great training information out there in the world. There are also many different schools of thought as well as various training systems out there. All of them have a lot of great information to offer. None of them are complete though. Not all of the training systems, or schools of thought, get along with each other. It is not our attempt to say that anyone's information is "wrong" or that our information is "right" or better than anyone else's training system. If anything, our goal is only to improve all training systems and modalities, to be ambassadors, if you will, to the other systems out there.

We honestly believe, and with good reason, that Bulletproof Fitness can enhance anyone's training modality. From Z-health, to

Functional Movement, to Gym Movement, we think our information presented here only enhances these systems.

From Tim:

Aside from that, I have always wanted to be capable of physically doing anything. All of us, if we are honest, have deep down inside wanted to be resilient, invincible, powerful, and strong. Mike and I believe we have found the secret to being bulletproof. The body is simply amazing. It is wonderfully designed. We were made to be perfect. As Mike has said, we have tried to outsmart what we were designed to do. We were made to move, to play, to live. Health is the key to being able to do all that you were designed to do. If all you want to do is just be a good parent, or volunteer at your local food shelter, or maybe you just want to be independent when you are 65, you need good health. What I mean is that if you truly want to enjoy your life to its fullest, you need to be healthy.

Good movement is the key to having good health. The better you move, the better your brain functions. The better your brain functions, the better you move. Midline crossing movements like the ones we have presented here are great tools for restoring our bodies' ability to move and function like they are meant to - perfectly.

I am not naive. I do not believe that the information we are presenting here is by any means complete. I know there is more wonder to be revealed. The more I think I learn, the more I realize I just don't know. Having said that, I believe the information we have presented here is a great place to start for developing a fully functional, capable body. The exercises in this book, if applied, can help you establish a great foundation, which is key to building a healthy structure.

As I said earlier, you have to put this information to the test. If you do not try anything in this book, you have no right to make any assumptions about what we are saying; good or bad. If you do desire to become bulletproof, give yourself a few months to engage in this material. Mike and I, along with some other friends, have been practicing this information for over a year now. Rome wasn't built in a day. It took time and consistent effort to build one of the most amazing empires the world has ever known. So it is too with the body. Becoming bulletproof is a process, a journey. Give yourself time to enjoy the journey.

From Mike

Hopefully the information we have presented will prove to be as useful to you as it has been to us. In addition, I hope your journey is as exciting and successful as ours has been. It's very easy to overlook that part: the journey. We always seem so focused on our destination that we lose sight of the experience along the way. My destination is complete athletic success. While I still haven't achieved that, my journey has provided me with a wealth of knowledge and a life long friend which is much more valuable to me than any physical reward I could take away.

So enjoy your journey and we hope this helps move you a bit closer to your physical destination.

Godspeed.

About the Authors

Mike and Tim

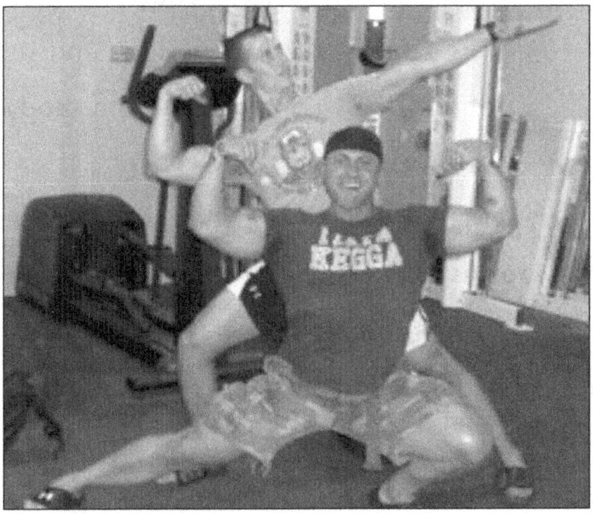

Mike and Tim's friendship began at a continuing educational seminar for trainers and therapist. From there, a conversation began that lead to the writings in this book.

Mike McNiff

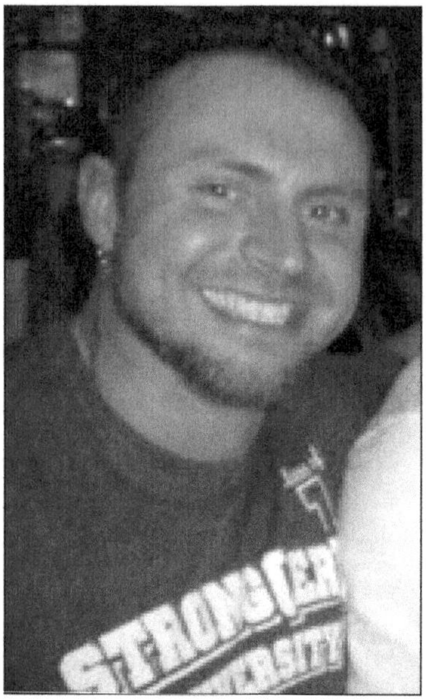

Mike began his education and coaching while rehabbing numerous injuries he received doing drug interdiction while on active duty. Upon his discharge, coaching became his full time passion. Mike has pursued continuing education with some of the top coaches and doctors in the country. Mike's education lead him to a focus in neurology and its effects on performance and body composition.

Mike is a former strength and conditioning coach for the wrestling team of John Hopkins University. He has also coached numerous levels of athletes from working mothers all the way to olympic athletes. Mike has even coached chiefs of staffs for members of congress.

Mike also has a competitive background in bodybuilding and strongman competitions.

Tim Anderson

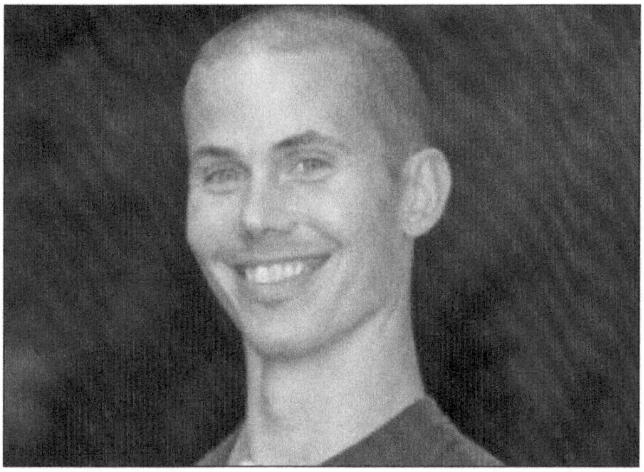

Tim is a husband of one and a father of two. He has been a certified personal trainer for over thirteen years and a professional firefighter for over twelve years.

Tim has had the fortune of learning from some of the brightest minds in the fitness industry. He has a passion for learning about all things health related and he loves sharing what he knows. Tim has had several training articles published and has even starred in a couple of physical training DVDs.

You can check Tim out at www.OPTfitness.net or email him at TAsfitness@earthlink.net.

References

1 Sally Goddard Blythe, *The Well Balanced Child* (Stroud: Hawthorne Press, 2005), p. 13.
2 Sally Goddard Blythe, *The Well Balanced Child* (Stroud: Hawthorne Press, 2005), p. xiv.
3 Carla Hannaford, *Smart Moves* (Salt Lake City: Great River Books, 2005), p. 48.
4 Carla Hannaford, *Smart Moves* (Salt Lake City: Great River Books, 2005), p. 32.
5 Carla Hannaford, *Smart Moves* (Salt Lake City: Great River Books, 2005), p. 28.
6 Sally Goddard Blythe, *The Well Balanced Child* (Stroud: Hawthorne Press, 2005), p. 176.
7 Sally Goddard Blythe, *The Well Balanced Child* (Stroud: Hawthorne Press, 2005), p. 23.
8 Barry Ross, *Underground Secrets to Faster Running* (BearPowered.com, 2005), p. 62.
9 Carla Hannaford, *Smart Moves* (Salt Lake City: Great River Books, 2005), p. 111.
10 Carla Hannaford, *Smart Moves* (Salt Lake City: Great River Books, 2005), p. 38.
11 Carla Hannaford, *Smart Moves* (Salt Lake City: Great River Books, 2005), p. 39.
12 Idem.
13 Sally Goddard Blythe, *The Well Balanced Child* (Stroud: Hawthorne Press, 2005), p. 13.
14 Carla Hannaford, *Smart Moves* (Salt Lake City: Great River Books, 2005), p. 38.
15 Carla Hannaford, *Smart Moves* (Salt Lake City: Great River Books, 2005), p. 49.
16 Carla Hannaford, *Smart Moves* (Salt Lake City: Great River Books, 2005), p. 39.
17 Sally Goddard Blythe, *The Well Balanced Child* (Stroud: Hawthorne Press, 2005), p. 18.
18 Sally Goddard Blythe, *The Well Balanced Child* (Stroud: Hawthorne Press, 2005), p. 19.
19 Idem.
20 Carla Hannaford, *Smart Moves* (Salt Lake City: Great River Books, 2005), p. 111.
21 Carla Hannaford, *Smart Moves* (Salt Lake City: Great River Books, 2005), p. 91.

22 Carla Hannaford, *Smart Moves* (Salt Lake City: Great River Books, 2005), p. 112.

23 Carla Hannaford, *Smart Moves* (Salt Lake City: Great River Books, 2005), p. 131.

24 Idem.

25 Idem.

26 Idem.

27 Carla Hannaford, *Smart Moves* (Salt Lake City: Great River Books, 2005), p. 112.

28 Idem.

29 Idem.

30 Sally Goddard Blythe, *The Well Balanced Child* (Stroud: Hawthorne Press, 2005), p. 185.

31 Gray Cook, *Secrets of Primitive Patterns* (Functional Movement DVD series)

32 Sally Goddard Blythe, *The Well Balanced Child* (Stroud: Hawthorne Press, 2005), p. 185.

33 www.functionalmovement.com!

34 Dan John, *Never Let Go* (Santa Cruz: On Target Publications, 2009), p. 123.

35 Gray Cook, *Movement* (Santa Cruz: On Target Publications, 2010), pps. 187 - 189.

36 www.functionalmovement.com

37 Gray Cook and Lee Burton, *Secrets of Primitive Patterns,* DVD (Functional Movement, 2008)

38 Gray Cook and Brett Jones, Secrets of the Shoulder, DVD (Functional Movement, 2006)

39 Pavel Tsatsouline, Power to the People (St. Paul: DragonDoor Publications, 1999), p. 64.

40 http://www.sciencebuddies.org/science-fair-projects/project_ideas/MatlSci_p021.shtml

41 Pavel Tsatsouline, *Power to the People* (St. Paul: Dragon Door Publications, 1999), p. 78.

42 Pavel Tsatsouline, *Power to the People* (St. Paul: Dragon Door Publications, 1999), p. 79.

43 Dan John, *Never Let Go* ((Santa Cruz: On Target Publications, 2009), p. 123.

44 Carla Hannaford, *Smart Moves* (Salt Lake City: Great River Books, 2005), p. 131.

CPSIA information can be obtained at www.ICGtesting.com
Printed in the USA
LVOW011926200513

334664LV00018B/593/P

9 781619 961968